CREDENTIALS COMMITTEE

Essentials Handbook

Richard A. Sheff, MD

Robert J. Marder, MD

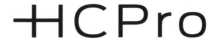

Credentials Committee Essentials Handbook is published by HCPro, Inc.

Copyright © 2012 HCPro, Inc.

Download the additional materials of this book at *www.hcpro.com/downloads/10552*

ISBN: 978-1-60146-945-8

HCPro, Inc., provides information resources for the healthcare industry. HCPro, Inc., is not affiliated in any way with The Joint Commission, which owns the JCAHO and Joint Commission trademarks.

Richard A. Sheff, MD, Author

Robert J. Marder, MD, Author

Katrina Gravel, Editorial Assistant

Elizabeth Jones, Editor

Erin Callahan, Associate
    Editorial Director

Mike Mirabello, Graphic Artist

Matt Sharpe, Production Supervisor

Shane Katz, Art Director

Jean St. Pierre, Senior Director of Operations

Advice given is general. Readers should consult professional counsel for specific legal, ethical, or clinical questions.

Arrangements can be made for quantity discounts. For more information, contact:

HCPro, Inc.

75 Sylvan Street, Suite A-101

Danvers, MA 01923

Telephone: 800-650-6787 or 781-639-1872

Fax: 800-639-8511

Email: *customerservice@hcpro.com*

Visit HCPro online at: *www.hcpro.com*
and *www.hcmarketplace.com*

Contents

Figure List.. vii

About the Authors... ix

Chapter 1: Principles of Effective Credentialing
and Privileging...1

Credentialing Principle #1:
Credentialing Exists to Protect Patients 1

Credentialing Principle #2:
No One Works Without a Ticket 3

Credentialing Principle #3:
Beware the Two Types of Credentialing Errors................................4

Credentialing Principle #4:
Credentialing Is Composed of Four Distinct Steps...........................5

Credentialing Principle #5:
Follow the Five Ps 8

Credentialing Principle #6: Excellent Credentialing
Requires Clear Criteria That Are Consistently Applied 9

Credentialing Principle #7: Place the Burden
on the Applicant 11

Credentialing Principle #8:
Treat Like Physicians in a Like Manner 12

Credentialing Principle #9: Before Granting Privileges,
Solve the Competency Equation...12

Credentialing Principle #10: To Match Competency
With Privileges, Use the Greeley Competency Triangle.................13

Credentialing Principle #11: Never Deny Membership or
Privileges, Except in Cases of Demonstrated Incompetence
or Unprofessional Conduct 15

Credentialing Principle #12:
Do Not Confuse Membership With Privileges.............................15

Chapter 2: Roles and Responsibilities of the
Credentials Committee 17

Power of the Pyramid..18

Medical Staff Functions..19

Definitions 21

Responsibilities of the Credentials Committee.............................22

Responsibilities of Credentials Committee Members....................27

Chapter 3: Focused Professional Practice
Evaluation for New Privileges..29

Defining FPPE...30

Evaluating Practitioner Care..33

Methods of On-Site Proctoring..34

Methods of Off-Site Proctoring 35

New Technology in Proctoring 35

Protecting Proctors From Liability...............................36

The Credentials Committee's Role in FPPE 38

Chapter 4: Privileges for New Technology 39

Follow the Five Ps 40

What Should the Technology Assessment Committee Do?...............41

Should the New Privileges Be Considered Core?...........42

Chapter 5: Effective, Data-Driven Reappointments...............45

Effective OPPE = Systematic Measurement
+ Evaluation + Follow-Through 47

Why Use a Physician Performance Feedback Report? 54

Chapter 6: Reappointment Challenges: Low- and No-volume Providers and Impaired and Aging Practitioners 57

Low- and No-Volume Practitioners 57

Impaired Practitioners 67

Aging Practitioners 69

Chapter 7: Privileging Disputes................................73

Chapter 8: The Credentials Committee's Role in Professional Conduct 79

How Does the Credentials Committee Handle
Conduct Issues as Part of the Appointment and
Reappointment Process? 80

Chapter 9: Effective Credentials Committee Meetings 83

Tip #1: Provide for Appropriate Leadership
and Membership 83

Tip #2: Spend Committee Time Wisely.........................85

Tip #3: Streamline Meetings by Eliminating Paper.......87

Tip #4: Don't Forget Surveillance Activities 87

Tip #5: Provide Committee Support 88

Figure List

Figure 1.1: The competency equation 13

Figure 2.1: When it comes to quality, who owns what? 18

Figure 2.2: The power of the pyramid 19

Figure 2.3: The medical staff's major functions................... 20

Figure 3.1: Sample FPPE plan for a newly trained
and board-certified cardiologist.. 31

Figure 3.2: Sample FPPE plan for a nurse-midwife 32

Figure 5.1: Quality indicators.. 49

Figure 5.2: One target, two performance levels 53

Figure 5.3: Two targets, three performance levels............. 53

Figure 6.1: Medical staff membership categories 61

Figure 6.2: Determining privilege level 66

About the Authors

Richard A. Sheff, MD

Richard A. Sheff, MD, is principal and chief medical officer with The Greeley Company, a division of HCPro, Inc., in Danvers, Mass. He brings more than 25 years of healthcare management and leadership experience to his work with physicians, hospitals, and healthcare systems across the country. With his distinctive combination of medical, healthcare, and management acumen, Dr. Sheff develops tailored solutions to the unique needs of physicians and hospitals. He consults, authors, and presents on a wide range of healthcare management and leadership issues, including governance, physician-hospital alignment, medical staff leadership development, ED call, peer review, hospital performance improvement, disruptive physician management, conflict resolution, physician employment and contracting, healthcare systems, service line management, hospitalist program optimization, patient safety and error reduction, credentialing, strategic planning, regulatory compliance, and helping physicians rediscover the joy of medicine.

Robert J. Marder, MD

Robert J. Marder, MD, is an advisory consultant and director of medical staff services with The Greeley Company, a division of HCPro, Inc., in Danvers, Mass. He brings more than 25 years of healthcare leadership and management experience to his work with physicians, hospitals, and healthcare organizations across the country. Dr. Marder's many roles in senior hospital medical administration and operations management in academic and community hospital settings make him uniquely qualified to assist physicians and hospitals in developing solutions for complex medical staff and hospital performance issues. He consults, authors, and presents on a wide range of healthcare leadership issues, including effective and efficient peer review, physician performance measurement and improvement, hospital quality measurement systems and performance improvement, patient safety/error reduction, and utilization management.

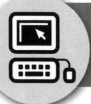

DOWNLOAD YOUR MATERIALS NOW

This handbook includes a customizable presentation that organizations can use to train physician leaders. The presentation complements the information provided in this handbook and can be downloaded at the following link:

www.hcpro.com/downloads/10552

Thank you for purchasing this product!

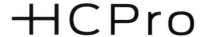

Principles of Effective Credentialing and Privileging

The credentials committee plays a critical role in the hospital, medical staff, and quality patient care. Yet medical staffs often assign members who lack adequate training to serve on the credentials committee. The intent of this book is to equip medical staff members with the information they need to serve effectively as members of the credentials committee. The following are 12 principles of credentialing that every credentials committee member should know.

Credentialing Principle #1: Credentialing Exists to Protect Patients

Why do hospitals credential practitioners? Credentialing exists to protect patients. Patients entrust their care to practitioners. When a practitioner turns to a patient or a family member and says, "I need to take you to the operating room. Don't worry—you're in good hands," the hospital must be confident that the practitioner is adequately trained and competent. That's what credentialing is about.

Patients and families in the community count on the credentials committee to do a good job on their behalf. When the credentials committee does its job poorly, patients are at risk for receiving poor-quality care and the hospital is at risk for litigation should a malpractice suit arise. Although credentialing requires following a specific set of rules to meet regulatory legal requirements and reduce liability, the credentialing processes should be flexible and physician-friendly.

Adequate credentialing should result in high-quality patient care and physician and hospital success. If a hospital overfocuses on any one of those areas to the neglect of the others, bad results will happen. For example, if a physician had been out on extended maternity leave and wanted to join the medical staff of ABC Hospital, but ABC's credentialing rules are so rigid as to not allow a physician on staff who has been out of practice for two years, the hospital might lose out on a qualified and competent physician. In this example, the hospital's efforts to provide high-quality patient care by limiting its staff affects physician success (the physician can't practice) and hospital success (the hospital loses referrals). A more flexible approach might be to require the physician to participate in additional training and undergo an extended period of focused professional practice evaluation before the medical staff grants her privileges.

Credentialing Principle #2: No One Works Without a Ticket

The second credentialing principle is that nobody works without a ticket. If a physician or an allied health professional (AHP) wants to provide inpatient care, that practitioner must be authorized to do so. Authorization can be carried out in one of three ways:

1. Medical staff privileges with quality monitoring through the medical staff. Practitioners are granted privileges for a scope of services, and the medical staff is responsible for ensuring that each practitioner does a good job.

2. Job description with supervision and annual performance evaluation. Employees of the hospital have job descriptions, and a manager supervises and evaluates their performance.

3. Contract with scope-of-service agreement. The hospital could have a contract with a scope of services agreement that defines what a practitioner or entity can do under that agreement and how performance will be monitored.

The idea of a ticket is to provide everyone who works in the hospital with a scope of responsibility, a clear chain of accountability, and ongoing quality monitoring.

Credentialing Principle #3: Beware the Two Types of Credentialing Errors

The third credentialing principle asks "How can the credentials committee make a mistake?" In general, there are two types of credentialing errors:

- **Information errors:** Information errors occur when information existed that would have affected a credentialing decision, but the medical staff was unaware. For example, if a physician was able to hide several malpractice cases, a license suspension, or a gap in training or experience, that would constitute an information error.

- **Decision errors:** Decision errors occur when the medical staff knows about malpractice cases, license suspensions, training gaps, etc., but fails to make a wise decision.

One of the credentials committee's responsibilities is to evaluate applicants for initial appointments, reappointments, and new privileges. The committee should find no gaps in training, the privileges requested should be typical for the physician's specialty, the National Practitioner Data Bank (NPDB) query should be clear, and references should all seem okay. The majority of files will sail through free and clear.

Occasionally, the committee will come across a file that sends up a red flag (e.g., a reference that leaves a line blank about the applicant's professional behavior, or all of the recommendations are excellent except for one low score regarding compliance with policies). In such a case, the credentials committee's job is to investigate the red flag and resolve the concern to the committee's satisfaction.

Credentialing Principle #4: Credentialing Is Composed of Four Distinct Steps

The fourth credentialing principle helps organize credentialing into four steps.

Step 1: Establish policies and rules

- Credentials committee, medical executive committee (MEC), and governing board

Step 2: Collect and summarize information

- Hospital management and medical staff leaders

Step 3: Evaluate and recommend

- Department chairs, MEC/credentials committee

Step 4: Grant or deny privileges

- Governing board or designated agent

Let's take a closer look at each of these steps.

Step 1: The credentials committee must establish the policies, procedures, and rules by which it will carry out credentialing functions. For example, what are the criteria for membership and privileges? What information will the committee request of applicants so it doesn't make an information error? What constitutes a completed application? How will the committee handle references? How will the medical staff handle turf battles?

The credentials committee doesn't establish policies, procedures, and rules on its own; it makes recommendations to the MEC, which in turn makes recommendations to the board.

Step 2: The credentials committee collects and summarizes information and creates a complete application file according to the processes defined in step one. This process is done primarily by the credentialing specialists in the medical staff services department, who are experts in how to query the NPDB, do primary source verification, and collect all the pieces of the puzzle.

Credentials committee members should not leave the entire process to the credentialing specialists. Rather, credentials committee members should contact the references on physicians' applications. In a small hospital, a committee member may be able to call every reference, but in a larger hospital, members may only be able to call references when an application raises a red flag. Whenever there is a need to clarify a problem encountered during the information collection process, it is the medical staff leader's job to call the references. Practitioners will tell another practitioner something they wouldn't put in writing.

Step 3: The credentials file is complete, and a department chair must evaluate that application according to the rules established during the first step. Once the evaluation is complete, the department chair makes a recommendation to the credentials committee. The credentials committee evaluates that recommendation and reviews the file independently. The credentials committee then makes a recommendation to the MEC, which reviews, revises, and discusses the credentials committee's recommendation and makes its own recommendation to the board.

Step 4: The governing board decides whether:

- The application will be approved

- All or some of the requested privileges will be granted, or all of them will be denied

- There will be a change to the physician's medical staff category

The Centers for Medicare & Medicaid Services' *Conditions of Participation* require that privileging decisions rest with the governing board. When physicians make decisions about the membership and privileges of fellow physicians, there's risk of breeching anticompetitive, antitrust, restraint-of-trade laws. That's why department chairs, credentials committees, and MECs make only recommendations; the board has the sole authority to grant or deny.

Credentialing Principle #5: Follow the Five Ps

Our Policy is to follow our Policy. In the absence of a Policy, our Policy is to develop a Policy.

At first, it seems this is a statement that only a bureaucrat could love, but it's a credentialing specialist's best friend. The Five Ps prevent hospitals from doing things on an ad hoc basis or treating practitioners prejudicially. When hospitals follow the Five Ps, they create policies and procedures and criteria and apply them consistently.

But what happens when a hospital is faced with a situation that it's never considered before, such as a new technology or privileging dispute, and therefore doesn't have a policy to guide it? Now what? Don't act. The Five Ps tell us that in the absence of a policy, our policy is to develop a policy. The hospital doesn't make a decision about that particular issue right away. Instead it conducts research and develops the necessary policy or criteria. Only then it is okay to return to the issue and make a decision.

The following list is a sample of the kinds of topics every hospital should have policies for.

- Criteria-based privileging

- New technology

- Privileging disputes

- Low-/no-volume practitioners

- Telemedicine

- Temporary privileges

- AHPs

- Expedited credentialing

These policies may exist independently, or they may be part of a credentialing policy and procedure manual. Some aspects may be in your bylaws.

Credentialing Principle #6: Excellent Credentialing Requires Clear Criteria That Are Consistently Applied

The sixth credentialing principle flows naturally from the Five Ps in that it prevents medical staffs from doing things without thinking them through and setting the criteria first. Medical staffs should not act in a prejudicial manner. A medical staff leader should never say, "I knew someone you worked with, and therefore you're a good person." Get away from the "good old boy" network. Credentialing is an objective process with criteria that need to be applied consistently. Two types of criteria apply to the credentialing process: membership criteria and privileging criteria.

Let's distinguish criteria for membership on the medical staff from criteria for privileging. Membership is a political question: Can the physician vote? Hold office? Constitute a quorum? Will the physician belong to the active, associate, courtesy, or emeritus staff category? The following list contains typical medical staff membership criteria.

- License

- Training

- Character and ethics

- Behavior

- Malpractice insurance

- Board certification

- Office/home location

Now let's consider privileging criteria. Privileges allow physicians to do specific tasks when treating patients. Privileging criteria include:

- License or certification

- Training (privilege specific)

- Experience

- Ability to perform requested privileges

- Evidence of current competence

Privileging criteria asks whether a physician's training is specific to the privileges he or she is requesting. What experience does the physician have doing that type of procedure or taking care of those types of patients? Is the physician competent to perform the privileges he or she is requesting? The competence question is the single most challenging aspect of credentialing, which brings us, in part, to the seventh principle.

Credentialing Principle #7: Place the Burden on the Applicant

Physicians must prove to the medical staff that they meet the medical staff's criteria.

If the credentials committee comes across a red flag in an application, it can ask for additional information, and the physician must answer the questions fully and honestly. Credentialing policies should reflect this requirement.

Credentialing Principle #8: Treat Like Physicians in a Like Manner

Sometimes during the credentialing process, a physician might say, "If you're asking for this additional information about me, don't you have to ask everyone else, too?" The answer is, "Not so fast." Credentialing policies should state that the credentials committee treats like physicians in a like manner. That is to say that physicians who have no gaps, questions, or red flags are treated similarly. The credentials committee drills down further for all physicians who represent red flags. Hospitals must place the burden on the applicant, so don't let an applicant tie you up in knots over "if you do this to me you have to do it to everyone else." Hospitals should treat physicians fairly, but that doesn't necessarily mean all physicians will be treated equally. If a physician falls into a category because of a red flag, the credentials committee must drill down and get additional information until it is satisfied.

Credentialing Principle #9: Before Granting Privileges, Solve the Competency Equation

Current competency, as we said, is the thorniest challenge. Before granting privileges, the credentials committee must solve the competency equation.

Figure 1.1   THE COMPETENCY EQUATION

> Current competency = Evidence that you've done it recently +
> Evidence that when you did it, you did it well

Through performance data, the credentials committee can find evidence that a physician has performed a procedure or task recently and performed it well.

Credentialing Principle #10: To Match Competency with Privileges, Use the Greeley Competency Triangle

To solve the competency equation, the Greeley Company recommends using the Greeley competency triangle. Avedis Donabedian, one of the great thinkers regarding quality, came up with Donabedian's Triangle, which says that quality is a function of three factors: structure, process, and outcome. The Greeley Company applied Donabedian's Triangle to competency and found that competency is a function of three elements: privilege delineation, eligibility criteria, and peer review results.

Privilege delineation: There are several ways we can delineate privileges. Medical staffs can choose to delineate privileges in a "laundry list," where every single task or procedure—from hemicolectomy to total colectomy to colectomy with colostomy—is listed. Some hospitals have moved to core privileging, where the privileging documents describe overall what a physician in a particular specialty does, and then pulls out specific procedures. Another way to delineate privileges is through competency clusters, where like privileges are grouped together. It's up to each medical staff to decide how it will delineate privileges.

Eligibility criteria: To develop eligibility criteria, the medical staff has to decide whether a practitioner must have had specific training to perform a procedure or must have performed the procedure successfully X number of times in the past two years. Perhaps the medical staff requires both.

If a physician does not meet the medical staff's eligibility criteria for a specific set of privileges, the medical staff should not process the practitioner's request for those privileges. Instead, the practitioner is ineligible to apply. When that happens, the medical staff should not deny the practitioner's application because a denial warrants a fair hearing and a report to the NPDB. (See the next section for more details about what to do in cases like this.)

Peer review results: Assuming that a physician is eligible to request privileges, the next step is to assess peer review results. For a new applicant, the medical staff should evaluate information regarding how the physician performed in other organizations; for reappointments, medical staffs must evaluate how well the physician functioned within organization.

Credentialing Principle #11: Never Deny Membership or Privileges, Except in Cases of Demonstrated Incompetence or Unprofessional Conduct

As previously stated, do not deny a physician's privileges unnecessarily. Denying membership or privileges is only appropriate in two cases: demonstrated incompetence or unprofessional conduct. Under any other circumstances, the physician is ineligible to apply for privileges. If the medical staff has evidence in the peer review results that a physician is providing poor-quality care and injuring patients or consistently acting in an unprofessional manner, the medical staff must deny his or her request for privileges.

Denying a physician's privileges gives him or her the right to a fair hearing and appeal. Fair hearings and appeals are time consuming and expensive, and tend to tear medical staffs apart. Establishing clear policies and eligibility criteria and using the competency triangle prevents medical staffs from denying membership or privileges except when a physician has demonstrated incompetence or unprofessional conduct.

Credentialing Principle #12: Do Not Confuse Membership with Privileges

As previously stated, criteria for membership are different than criteria for privileges. Membership is a political process, and the medical staff category a physician belongs to will determine whether a physician can vote, hold office, or constitute a quorum. Privileges are what the hospital allows a physician to do while treating patients.

These 12 principles will allow you to credential and privilege physicians in the best interest of patient care while also seeking to achieve physician success and hospital success in a balanced and effective manner.

Roles and Responsibilities of the Credentials Committee

There is often a disconnect between what the medical staff bylaws say the credentials committee members should do and what they actually do. The purpose of this chapter is to explain the roles and responsibilities of the members of the credentials committee.

The organized medical staff was created in the early 20th century to oversee and improve the quality of care on behalf of a governing board. Since the 1980s, the medical executive committee (MEC) has largely taken over that function. The MEC is responsible for overseeing the performance of all practitioners who are granted privileges. Practitioners can include not only physicians, but also dentists, oral and maxillofacial surgeons, psychologists, podiatrists, and allied health professionals who are privileged through the organized medical staff. The chief executive officer (CEO) oversees the performance of the system or the hospital as a whole and the performance of employees within that system.

Figure 2.1

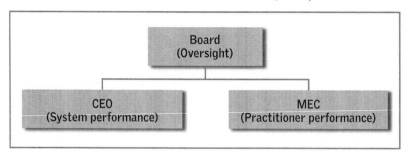

WHEN IT COMES TO QUALITY, WHO OWNS WHAT?

Power of the Pyramid

The late Howard Kurz introduced his pyramid model to the American College of Physician Executives more than two decades ago. For those of you not familiar with this model, the purpose of the pyramid is to enhance physician performance by increasing efficiency and decreasing conflict, thus helping every physician and practitioner be the best that he or she can be.

The medical staff should spend the greatest amount of time on the foundation layers of the pyramid so that, hopefully, it will never have to take corrective action (see figure 2.2). The base of this pyramid is credentialing and privileging. The best way to address a performance issue is at appointment and reappointment. Once a physician gets through the door, any problems that physician brings with him or her is the medical staff's to own for up to the next two years. The other layers of the pyramid have more to do with the peer review process.

Figure 2.2   THE POWER OF THE PYRAMID

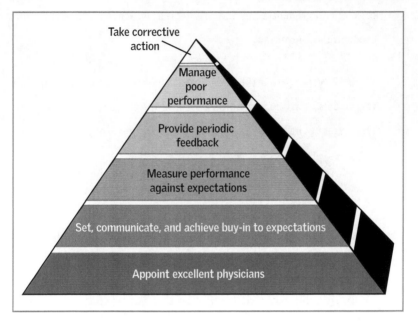

Medical Staff Functions

To make the foundation layers of the pyramid work, it's important to understand the medical staff's major functions.

- MEC (Governance)

- Credentials committee (Credentialing)

- Medical staff quality committee (Peer Review)

The MEC is the governing structure of the organized medical staff. The other two major functions of the medical staff include peer review, which usually goes through the medical staff quality committee, and credentialing and privileging, which is a function of the credentials committee.

Figure 2.3 shows that the department chairs are responsible to both the medical staff quality committee and the credentials committee. Department chairs are responsible for recommending:

- Indicators, quality metrics, and targets to the quality committee

- Candidates for membership or privileges to the credentials committee

- Eligibility criteria for membership and privileges to the credentials committee

Figure 2.3   **THE MEDICAL STAFF'S MAJOR FUNCTIONS**

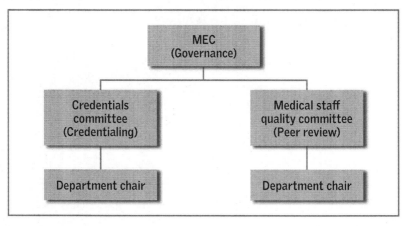

Definitions

Credentialing

One of the medical staff's major functions is to credential every physician who applies to the medical staff. But what does that mean? Credentialing is the verification of credentials to practice medicine, which also includes qualifications to serve as a member of the organized medical staff (e.g., training, background, experience, character, ethics, behavior, and current competence). Whenever feasible, information should be verified from the original or primary source of the credential (e.g., the institution where a physician completed his or her residency, the medical school the practitioner graduated from). Credentialing is time- and labor-intensive but is an important medical staff responsibility.

Privileging

Privileging is the act of deciding what a provider is allowed to do to a patient. Every order written, procedure performed, or consultation made requires a privilege. The challenge is to match the privileges the medical staff grants to a practitioner to the practitioner's demonstrated current competence.

The Joint Commission requires that privileging be an objective, evidence-based process. In the past, the credentials committee typically met every two years and asked if there was any negative information about an applicant, either for appointment or for reappointment. Today, The Joint Commission wants medical staffs to measure performance continuously, not just at two-year intervals.

Responsibilities of the Credentials Committee

First and foremost, the credentials committee's responsibility is to develop, recommend, and implement policies and procedures to continuously improve all credentialing and privileging activities. If the committee does not have a clear process to follow, it may not be able to manage charged situations efficiently. For example, credentials committees should have processes for managing aging practitioners, impaired practitioners, low-/no-volume practitioners, and privileges for new technology.

Second, the credentials committee is responsible for recommending to the MEC criteria for all privileges in each specialty after reviewing recommendations from the relevant department chairs. Department chairs may offer conflicting recommendations, so it is up to the credentials committee to make the best recommendation to the MEC.

Third, the credentials committee is in charge of reconciling differences between departments regarding criteria for cross-specialty privileges. For example, gastroenterologists may feel that general surgeons must perform more endoscopies to prove their competence because they do not specialize in endoscopies, but the general surgeons feel that they should only have to perform as many endoscopies as the gastroenterologists do. These can be heated debates, and it is up to the credentials committee to make the call.

Fourth, the credentials committee is responsible for recommending the process for establishing practitioner competency for all newly granted privileges based on department chairs' recommendations. In other words, the credentials committee should determine when each focused professional practice evaluation (FPPE) process has been adequately completed (although the department chairs will manage the process within their clinical departments). The medical staff should make the FPPE process as flexible as possible, and both the department chairs and the credentials committee should have the right to extend or shorten FPPE as needed.

Further responsibilities of the credentials committee include reviewing and recommending all applicants and reapplicants for membership on the medical staff, including the assignment of a medical staff category. Finally, the credentials committee should review and recommend actions on all requests for privileges from eligible practitioners.

How to evaluate a credentials file

Another responsibility of the credentials committee is to evaluate credentials files and recommend action on all initial appointments and reappointments after reviewing recommendations from the appropriate department chairs. The credentials committee has the right to modify, accept, or reject department chairs' recommendations.

Credentials committee members must evaluate applications with a keen eye for red flags. Does a red flag mean that a practitioner is not qualified? No. It just means that that the credentials committee needs to evaluate that red flag until it determines whether it is a substantial concern. Examples of typical red flags include:

- Gaps in training or practice

- Previous corrective action

- Professional competence or conduct issues

- Incomplete or inaccurate information provided on the application

- Unusual requests based on background and training

- Multiple changes in practice sites

- That "funny feeling" that an applicant doesn't measure up

The credentials committee must evaluate the references, particularly those that are less than stellar, incomplete, or contain unanswered questions. If a reference is incomplete, the credentials committee must put the burden on the applicant to complete the reference.

Credentials committee members should call references to get a complete picture of a physician applicant. If a reference asks, "Is this on the record or off the record?" always answer that it is on the record. Carefully document the content of the conversation. If the individual won't talk over the telephone, put the burden on the applicant to ensure a complete reference with the necessary information.

Chiefs of staff and members of credentials committees have reported that the telephone calls to individual references have the greatest impact, despite that making those calls is so time consuming. People will say things verbally that they will never put in writing, and that information is highly effective and useful.

Another important strategy for reviewing credentials files is to risk-stratify all applications. The recommendation 1, or R-1, category is for clean applicants without any red flags. The R-2 category refers to applicants with minor issues that do not require ongoing monitoring. R-3 applicants have significant issues that require ongoing monitoring.

The MEC and the board generally appreciate a ranking system because the board is concerned that it is getting incomplete information from both the credentials committee and the MEC. A ranking system helps to assure them that the credentials committee is, in fact, looking for different types of applicants that may be of greater risk than others. For all R-2 and R-3 candidates, the credentials committee should document the basis of its recommendation.

- Evaluate references

  - Less than stellar

  - Incomplete/unanswered questions

  - Read between the lines

- Review calls to references

  - "Is this on the record or off the record?"

  - Is the conversation adequately documented?

- When a red flag is identified, drill down to resolve the concern to the committee's satisfaction

- Risk-stratify the application

  - R-1: Clean applicants without red flags

  - R-2: Applicants with minor issues that do not require ongoing monitoring

  - R-3: Applicants with significant issues that require ongoing monitoring

- For all R-2 and R-3 applicants, document the basis of the committee's recommendations

The MEC and the governing board will almost always agree with the credentials committee's recommendation based on the credentials committee's expertise in credentialing.

Responsibilities of Credentials Committee Members

Individual credentials committee members are responsible for the following duties:

- Regularly attending committee meetings

- Reviewing assigned credentials files prior to the meeting so as to not waste meeting time with routine activities

- Complying with the medical staff's conflict-of-interest and confidentiality policies

- Continuously seeking to enhance knowledge and understanding of credentialing

- Always acting in good faith, without bias, and in the best interests of patient care

Credentials committee members should place the interests of patients, the hospital, the medical staff, and the community first, and not have any decisions driven by a personal agenda.

Focused Professional Practice Evaluation for New Privileges

One may think that focused professional practice evaluation (FPPE) is solely the peer review or quality committee's responsibility, but the credentials committee must understand how it is performed and how to evaluate the results if the committee is going to make wise credentialing and privileging recommendations to the medical executive committee (MEC).

FPPE is a term coined by The Joint Commission. The Joint Commission uses the same term to describe two different activities. One type of FPPE is used to evaluate new privileges, whether a practitioner is applying to the medical staff for the first time or is already a medical staff member requesting new privileges. The second type of FPPE is to evaluate the performance of existing medical staff members when the data gathered during ongoing professional practice evaluation (OPPE) indicate a problem. The second type of FPPE is handled by the peer review committee; it is not a function of the credentials committee.

Defining FPPE

FPPE is a Joint Commission requirement, but your organization does not need to be Joint Commission–accredited to conduct FPPE. When a practitioner joins the medical staff, the medical staff has made its best decision based on evidence of the care the practitioner has provided in other organizations. The credentials committee can't guarantee the practitioner's performance; it is just doing its best to predict his or her performance. Remember: The best predictor of future behavior is past behavior. Once a practitioner has joined the organization, the medical staff must measure and evaluate whether it has made a good decision.

FPPE is a more timely, in-depth measurement of the quality of care provided by practitioners who:

- Are new to the medical staff (broad)

- Want to do something new outside of their core privileges (less broad)

- Have concerns raised through OPPE that need to be verified (narrow)

FPPE is not one-size-fits-all. Each specialty is different, and each applicant is different. Therefore, the medical staff must customize FPPE to the applicant's circumstances. FPPE does not require that every practitioner is concurrently proctored (concurrent proctoring requires one physician to watch another physician perform the requested privileges). Rather, some practitioners may simply require chart review, or they may be required to review their care plan with another practitioner before treating a patient (prospective review). Figures 3.1 and 3.2 provide examples of FPPE plans for applicants in different specialties.

Years ago, medical staffs simply placed all new applicants into a provisional category of the medical staff. A practitioner joined the staff, waited two years, and if nothing went wrong, he or she was promoted to the active medical staff category. FPPE is a more proactive approach to ensuring that only competent practitioners are on the medical staff. The purpose of conducting FPPE early on

Figure 3.1

SAMPLE FPPE PLAN FOR A NEWLY TRAINED AND BOARD-CERTIFIED CARDIOLOGIST

Skill being evaluated	Activity being evaluated	Method for evaluating the activity
Cognitive skills	10 cases of varied diagnoses, including MI, infarction, CHF, etc. (covering privileges granted)	Retrospective review
Procedural skills	Two diagnostic and four interventional catheterizations	Concurrent proctoring
Projected time frame: Within 90 days of being granted clinical privileges		

Figure 3.2

Sample FPPE Plan for a Nurse Midwife

Skill being evaluated	Activity being evaluated	Method for evaluating the activity
Cognitive skills	Manage midwifery elements of (n) moderate risk cases after consultation with physician	Retrospective review
	Manage midwifery elements of (n) high-risk cases after consultation with physician	Prospective review
Procedural skills	Deliver (n) patients and manage (n) infants at delivery	Concurrent proctoring
	Perform (n) amniotomy procedures	Concurrent proctoring
	Perform (n) episiotomy and repair procedures	Concurrent proctoring
	Perform (n) vacuum extractions	Concurrent proctoring
Projected time frame: Within 90 days of being granted clinical privileges		

is not to prove that a practitioner is bad; it is so that if the medical staff catches issues early, it can provide feedback and give practitioners a chance to succeed in the organization. The medical staff can also decide fairly quickly if it has made a mistake in the credentialing and privileging process.

FPPE requires follow-through, so that if the medical staff finds a concern, it can provide feedback to the practitioner. This is why FPPE is really owned by the credentials committee: The credentials committee makes the original thorough assessment and decision based on the recommendation of the department chair.

Evaluating Practitioner Care

There are two types of care a practitioner can provide: cognitive and procedural. Cognitive care involves listening, thinking about, and diagnosing, whereas procedural care involves performing procedures. The credentials committee must evaluate both the cognitive and procedural aspects of care.

In the past, medical staffs would identify charts that fell outside the norm and give them a "sniff test" to determine whether the standard of care was met on a subjective basis. That kind of evaluation creates a lot of conflict. Physicians feel they are treated unfairly, and the evaluation is prone to inter-rater variation. Using indicators is a fair, objective means of evaluating practitioner performance.

It is important for credentials committee members to understand the three types of indicators:

- Rules: standard ways of taking care of patients (e.g., no unsafe abbreviations, no acting in an unprofessional manner)

- Rates: a numerator, a denominator, and a target; the goal is to determine how performance compares to the target

- Reviews: reviews include proctoring, not just chart reviews

If a practitioner breaks a rule, the medical staff should provide him or her with automatic feedback and trend his or her performance over time. If a rate is trending in the wrong direction, the credentials committee should constantly evaluate it and refer the physician to the department chair. If you have an unusual event or if proctoring unearths a problem, the credentials committee must act immediately to provide the physician feedback and get to the root of the problem.

Methods of On-Site Proctoring

There are three types of proctoring:

- Prospective: when a practitioner presents a care plan to the credentials committee, and the credentials committee decides whether it is a good approach

- Concurrent: when a practitioner directly observes another practitioner in action

- Retrospective: when a practitioner has already provided care for a patient, and now the credentials committee reviews it through case reviews, charts, or video

Methods of Off-Site Proctoring

The medical staff may not be able to proctor a physician on site because, for example, the physician provides the majority of care at another facility. In such cases, it may be necessary for the medical staff to perform off-site proctoring, of which there are two types:

- Reciprocal: This uses concurrent work completed at another organization or institution as a tool for evaluating the applicant.

- Preemptive: This leverages proctoring results from the physician's original institution prior to granting privileges at your organization.

New Technology in Proctoring

Medical staffs should take advantage of new technologies to help them perform FPPE, including teleproctoring, procedure recording, and simulation.

Teleproctoring. If an organization does not have a practitioner on staff with the appropriate expertise to evaluate a practitioner who is using a new technology or new privileges, the medical staff can teleproctor. Using live video streaming, a proctor can observe a practitioner in real-time and evaluate the quality of the procedure that the practitioner is performing.

Procedure recording. Medical staffs can record a practitioner performing a procedure and have a proctor retrospectively evaluate it.

Simulation. The field is in its infancy, but technology is improving so that practitioners can use a simulator to test all kinds of situations and procedures. It has proven effective in aeronautics and aerospace, and now there will be more simulation in medicine as well.

Protecting Proctors From Liability

FPPE may result in a number of potential dilemmas. Medical staffs should establish in their policies the type of liability coverage and protections for proctoring physicians.

Medical staffs must decide their comfort level. For example, is it the role of the proctor to intervene if a case goes wrong, or is the proctor simply there to observe the procedure? What happens if the medical staff wants to discontinue, prolong, or shorten FPPE for a particular physician? What is the legal liability related to the proctoring reports? Will reports have some status that can then be used if a patient or physician sues the physician or the hospital later? Are there conflicts of interest between the proctor and the practitioner being proctored? What do you tell patients and staff when a practitioner is being proctored?

Potential dilemmas regarding FPPE include:

- Liability coverage and protection for the proctor

- Intervention if the case does not go well

- Stopping, prolonging, or shortening FPPE

- Legal liability of proctoring reports

- Conflicts of interest

- Conflict between proctor and practitioner undergoing FPPE

- What to tell patients and staff when a practitioner is being proctored

Your FPPE and conflict-of-interest policies should address each of those dilemmas. Your FPPE policy should include:

- What triggers FPPE

- Who triggers FPPE

- What does FPPE look like for each clinical service or specialty

- Who determines when it is complete

- Who reports the findings to MEC

The Credentials Committee's Role in FPPE

The credentials committee's role in FPPE for new members and new privileges include:

- Creating and continuously improving the FPPE policy and procedure over time to improve efficiency and effectiveness

- Reviewing and modifying the FPPE plan for each new practitioner and each new privilege as recommended by the department chair

- Reviewing and evaluating all reports on the progress and completion of each FPPE plan

- Determining when an FPPE plan is complete

- Determining whether the department chair is able to increase or decrease the number of cases to be reviewed or change the FPPE plan for practitioners

- Determining what types of reports the MEC will require.

- Addressing how to deal with conflicts of interest or complaints of bias.

Regardless of whether an institution is Joint Commission–accredited, the credentials committee's job is to make sure that new practitioners or practitioners requesting new privileges or technologies are evaluated in a timely manner with timely follow-through so that each physician is providing the best possible care.

Privileges for New Technology

A practitioner informs the medical staff president that he would like to schedule one of his patients for a new procedure using new equipment. He has already arranged for a representative from the company that manufactures the equipment to deliver it to the facility within the next week. What is the first question the medical staff president should ask?

Although medical staff leaders may think that the first question to ask is whether the practitioner has privileges for the new procedure, the question that should come first is "Is this procedure within the scope of services this hospital provides?" This is a decision that will have to go through the MEC and the governing board because, ultimately, the governing board must determine what privileges and services the hospital offers. Once that question is answered, it's time to delve into whether the practitioner is competent and qualified to perform the new procedure.

Follow the Five Ps

When you're dealing with any difficult process, particularly one that has political and economic implications for the facility, such as new technology, the best thing to do is to follow the Five Ps: *Our policy is to follow our policy. In the absence of a policy, our policy is to create a policy.*

If the medical staff doesn't have a policy regarding how to privilege new technologies, the best thing to do is to call a timeout and create such a policy and procedure.

A new technology policy should spell out the roles of the following three committees:

- Technology assessment committee (ad hoc subcommittee of the credentials committee or a hospital committee with physician representation)

- Institutional review board (IRB)

- Ethics committee

Assessing technology is more complicated than it seems. It's not just about whether the hospital should offer the service, or even about what the eligibility criteria should be for practitioners who are going to exercise this new clinical privilege. It also has to do with whether the hospital has the infrastructure to safely offer the service. If so, what quality metrics will it establish, what equipment will the practitioners need, and what training will the hospital provide?

An IRB is helpful if the new technology is part of an experimental procedure, modality, or treatment. Some of these new technologies will involve ethical considerations, particularly concerning prolonging life, which the ethics committee should weigh in on.

What Should the Technology Assessment Committee Do?

The new technology assessment committee should debate the following questions.

Will this new procedure be within the hospital's scope of service?

- Is it safe and effective, or is it still experimental?

- Is it appropriate for the scope and complexity of the institution?

- Is it approved for reimbursement?

- What additional hospital resources will be required?

- Will the hospital receive reimbursement that covers the additional costs?

If the answers to the above set of questions are yes, the committee should move on to the next set of questions.

What will be the privileging criteria for the new procedure?

- Is it covered under an exclusive contract?

- Does it require the same knowledge and skills as other existing privileges?

- Is there already a generally recognized standard for eligibility regarding training and experience?

- What criteria have other institutions already developed?

- Will multiple specialties be interested?

Hospitals have the right to sign exclusive contracts with practitioners and groups of practitioners, and if the new privilege is covered under an exclusive agreement, other practitioners may not be eligible to apply for it. If this causes political strife, the credentials committee may need to negotiate with management, the board, and the practitioners to decide whether to carve out the privilege from an exclusive contract that is already in effect.

Should the New Privileges Be Considered Core?

As explained in Chapter 3, some hospitals use "laundry list" privileges, whereas others group core privileges together. If the medical staff uses core privileges, the credentials committee must identify whether the new privileges require the same knowledge and skills as existing privileges. If so, the new privilege can probably be included in the core privileges. If not, the credentials committee may need to create additional criteria outside of the core. The committee can also create different eligibility criteria based on different clinical specialties.

Remember credentialing principle #7: Place the burden on the applicant. If a practitioner wants unique privileges or to introduce new technology, ask the practitioner to gather the information on your behalf. Applicants often won't have a problem gathering this data if they really are interested in achieving some kind of financial return and providing enhanced services to their patients as a result of the new technology.

Effective, Data-Driven Reappointments

In addition to vetting new medical staff applicants, the credentials committee is also responsible for ensuring that the existing members of the staff are qualified and competent to perform the privileges they have been granted. Reappointment should not be a rubber-stamping process; rather, data should drive the decision to reappoint a physician.

Let's go back to the pyramid (see Chapter 2) and ask where reappointment falls. Theoretically, the answer could be in every single layer. For example, the reappointment period can be the perfect time to set, communicate, and achieve buy-in to performance expectations to meet a particular goal, such as improved patient satisfaction scores. It's an opportunity to create a complete profile of a practitioner's performance based on ongoing evaluations or provide feedback indicating that a practitioner is not meeting expectations (although it should not be the first time the practitioner is hearing this news).

The question that unfortunately applies too often at reappointment is "Has this practitioner made enough mistakes in the past two years to warrant eliminating membership or privileges?" This is not a performance-improving approach to reappointment. If the medical staff is waiting until a practitioner has made enough mistakes to jeopardize his or her privileges or membership, it's too late. The medical staff should have been gathering and analyzing performance data all along and communicating the results to the practitioner before it got to this point. Practitioners can become defensive, and threatening their privileges is a high-stakes game.

Here's a way to think about reappointment: The credentials committee should be evaluating physicians' performance on an ongoing basis. Reappointment should simply be a punctuation mark in that ongoing process; it should not be the first time the credentials committee addresses a performance issue, sets performance expectations, provides feedback, or manages poor performance. The credentials committee should tackle those issues when they arise.

The Joint Commission has raised the bar by creating a standard that says, "The decision to grant or deny a privilege(s) and/or to renew an existing privilege(s) is an objective, evidenced-based process" (MS.06.01.05). Even if your facility isn't Joint Commission–accredited, the credentialing, privileging, and appointment processes should still be objective and evidence-based. That is where focused professional practice evaluation (FPPE) and ongoing professional practice evaluation (OPPE) come into the picture.

The credentialing process is a "customer" of the peer review process. Remember the Greeley competency triangle in Chapter 1, which consists of privilege delineation, eligibility criteria, and peer review results. At reappointment, the credentials committee must review peer review results (i.e., FPPE and OPPE data) to determine whether a practitioner is performing well.

Tip: The credentials committee can ask the peer review committee or medical executive committee for more information if it is not getting the data it needs to make an informed decision.

Effective OPPE = Systematic Measurement + Evaluation + Follow-Through

If FPPE is defined as timely measurement, evaluation, and follow-through, OPPE is about systematic measurement, evaluation, and follow-through. It does not have to be compressed in time, such as during the first couple of months after a practitioner joins the medical staff or requests new privileges. OPPE is the medical staff's ongoing radar screen for evaluating the quality of every practitioner's performance.

To interpret FPPE and OPPE data, the credentials committee must understand how quality indicators are used.

Quality indicators are based on performance expectations. The Joint Commission has adopted what the Accreditation Council for Graduate Medical Education has called general competencies, which are dimensions of practitioner performance. The late Howard Kurz, who developed the pyramid approach discussed in Chapter 2, used a different set of dimensions for practitioner performance. Either one is fine to use, as every element of one framework exists in the other; the two frameworks simply provide different ways of organizing performance expectations. Figure 5.1 outlines both sets of quality indicators.

Once the credentials committee has established performance expectations through a competency framework, establish indicators for each category of the framework. For example, if the medical staff has chosen the Greeley framework, an indicator of citizenship might be that a physician attends five medical staff meetings per year. The Joint Commission will likely settle for a couple of indicators in several different categories, but the best practice is to have indicators in each of the categories of physician performance.

The next step is to set performance targets. If practitioner performance is compared to a target, how many targets are necessary?

Figure 5.1

QUALITY INDICATORS

Greeley/ACPE framework

Technical Quality of Care: Skill and judgment related to effectiveness and appropriateness in performing the clinical privileges granted as evidenced by the following:

- Achieve patient outcomes that meet or exceed generally accepted medical staff standards as defined by comparative data, medical literature, and results of peer review evaluations
- Use sound clinical judgment based on patient information, available scientific evidence, and patient preferences to develop and carry out patient management plans
- Use evidence-based guidelines when available as recommended by the appropriate specialty in selecting the most effective and appropriate approaches to diagnosis and treatment

Quality of Service: Ability to meet the customer service needs of patients and other caregivers as evidenced by the following:

- Demonstrate caring and respectful behaviors when interacting with patients and their families
- Respond promptly to requests for patient care needs

Peer and Coworker Relationships: Interpersonal interactions with colleagues, hospital staff, and patients as evidenced by the following:

- Act in a professional, respectful manner at all times to enhance a spirit of cooperation and mutual respect and trust among members of the patient care team

Figure 5.1

Citizenship: Participation and cooperation with medical staff responsibilities as evidenced by the following:

- Review your individual and specialty data for all dimensions of performance and use this data for self-improvement to continuously improve patient care
- Participate in emergency room call coverage as determined by medical staff policy

Patient Safety/Patient Rights: Cooperation with patient safety and rights, rules, and procedures as evidenced by the following:

- Participate in the hospital's efforts and policies to maintain a patient safety culture, reduce medical errors, meet National Patient Safety Goals, and improve quality
- Communicate clearly with other physicians and caregivers, patients, and patients' families through appropriate oral and written methods to ensure accurate transfer of information
- Respect patients' rights by discussing unanticipated adverse outcomes and by not discussing patient care information and issues in public settings

Resource Utilization: Effective and efficient use of hospital clinical resources as evidenced by the following:

- Strive to provide cost-effective quality patient care by cooperating with efforts to manage the use of valuable patient care resources

The Joint Commission/ACGME framework

Patient Care: Practitioners are expected to provide patient care that is compassionate, appropriate, and effective for the promotion of health, for the

Figure 5.1

QUALITY INDICATORS (CONT.)

prevention of illness, for the treatment of disease, and at the end of life as evidenced by the following:

- Achieve patient outcomes that meet or exceed generally accepted medical staff standards as defined by comparative data and targets, medical literature, and results of peer review evaluations
- Use sound clinical judgment based on patient information, available scientific evidence, and patient preferences to develop and carry out patient management plans
- Demonstrate caring and respectful behaviors when interacting with patients and their families

Medical Knowledge: Practitioners are expected to demonstrate knowledge of established and evolving biomedical, clinical, and social sciences, and the application of their knowledge to patient care and the education of others, as evidenced by the following:

- Use evidence-based guidelines when available, as recommended by the appropriate specialty, in selecting the most effective and appropriate approaches to diagnosis and treatment

Practice-Based Learning and Improvement: Practitioners are expected to be able to use scientific evidence and methods to investigate, evaluate, and improve patient care as evidenced by the following:

- Review your individual and specialty data for all general competencies, and use this data for self-improvement to continuously improve patient care

Interpersonal and Communication Skills: Practitioners are expected to demonstrate interpersonal and communication skills that enable them to establish

Figure 5.1   Quality indicators (cont.)

and maintain professional relationships with patients, families, and other members of healthcare teams as evidenced by the following:

- Communicate clearly with other physicians and caregivers, patients, and patients' families through appropriate oral and written methods to ensure accurate transfer of information

Professionalism: Practitioners are expected to demonstrate behaviors that reflect a commitment to continuous professional development, ethical practice, an understanding and sensitivity to diversity, and a responsible attitude toward their patients, their profession, and society as evidenced by the following:

- Act in a professional, respectful manner at all times to enhance a spirit of cooperation and mutual respect and trust among members of the patient care team
- Respond promptly to requests for patient care needs
- Respect patients' rights by discussing unanticipated adverse outcomes and by not discussing patient care information and issues in public settings
- Participate in emergency room call coverage as determined by medical staff policy

Systems-Based Practice: Practitioners are expected to demonstrate both an understanding of the contexts and systems in which healthcare is provided, and the ability to apply this knowledge to improve and optimize healthcare, as evidenced by the following:

- Strive to provide cost-effective quality patient care by cooperating with efforts to manage the use of valuable patient care resources
- Participate in the hospital's efforts and policies to maintain a patient safety culture, reduce medical errors, meet National Patient Safety Goals, and improve quality

Figure 5.2   ONE TARGET, TWO PERFORMANCE LEVELS

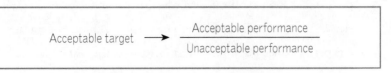

Figure 5.2 shows one target, which creates two performance levels. Above the target is acceptable performance, and below it is unacceptable performance. Using one target can have a negative effect on the medical staff culture because it is considered to be the "bad apples" approach. Rather than identifying opportunities for improvement, it focuses on poor performance. When using a "pass or fail" approach to peer review, practitioners tend to set the bar low because they don't want their peers to fall below the target. This approach does not drive excellence.

Alternatively, setting two targets, a "good enough" or "acceptable" target and an "excellent" target, creates three categories of performance (see figure 5.3). Clearly, performance data that falls above the excellent target is excellent performance. In the middle is acceptable performance, and below that needs follow-up.

Figure 5.3   TWO TARGETS, THREE PERFORMANCE LEVELS

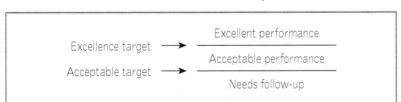

Practitioners are often overachievers, and when they see someone performing at an excellent level when they themselves are not, physicians often naturally improve. This creates a culture of continuous performance improvement. It recognizes the highest level of performance while stimulating those in the acceptable target range to self-improve. It also addresses potentially poor performance.

Why Use a Physician Performance Feedback Report?

Once the medical staff has established a competency framework and performance targets, it's time to start measuring and compiling performance data. As stated previously, physicians tend to be overachievers, and seeing their performance data on paper often spurs them toward self-improvement. Thus, physician performance report cards are a great way to drive physicians toward excellence. However, report cards have several other purposes as well:

- Set expectations of performance

- Recognize good performance

- Identify individual opportunities for improving practitioner performance

- Allow practitioners the opportunity to self-correct

- Provide a basis for dialog between medical staff leaders and practitioners regarding performance

- Provide a basis for managing poor performance

- Indicate red flags during the reappointment process

Again, when a practitioner receives a report card, it should not be the first time he or she is learning about his or her performance. Ideally, the peer review committee provides the physician with OPPE data throughout the year.

The peer review process allows the credentials committee to have performance data at the time of reappointment. Applying the Greeley competency triangle to the reappointment process will help the credentials committee match demonstrated competence with privileges at reappointment.

Reappointment Challenges:
Low- and No-Volume Providers and
Impaired and Aging Practitioners

Credentialing a practitioner with no red flags is already a pains-
taking process, so what about practitioners who present challenges,
such as those who are impaired, aging, or simply don't treat enough
patients at the hospital to generate adequate performance data?
These types of practitioners require special treatment during the
credentialing and reappointment processes.

Low- and No-volume Practitioners

More hospitals are faced with a growing number of low- and no-
volume practitioners: practitioners who don't treat enough patients
at the hospital for the medical staff to gather adequate performance
data. The number of low- and no-volume practitioners is growing
for several reasons.

- Changing financial incentives. It is generally more lucra-
  tive for practitioners to spend the majority of their time in
  their office practices than at the hospital. It used to be that

physicians made the majority of their livelihood taking care of hospitalized patients. That is becoming less of the norm today.

- Increased performance expectations from external regulators. External evaluators are enforcing strict performance expectations, including one that requires every practitioner with intensive care unit privileges to be qualified to exercise those privileges and not just be there to take call.

- Rapid growth of hospitalists. Hospitalists are replacing private practice physicians who no longer wish to practice in the hospital, and the trend has a cyclical effect. The more hospitalists there are, the more private practice physicians leave the hospital setting.

- Increased liability.

- Lifestyle preferences. Generation X and Generation Y want to do a better job balancing their personal and professional lives than generations past have. Office practices allow them to do that.

- Payer requirements. Payers are requiring practitioners to have current clinical competence and are properly credentialed and privileged to perform privileges, and for some practitioners, giving up privileges is simpler than going through the credentialing and privileging process to do a procedure five times in a year.

Strategic and competency goals

When deciding whether to allow low- and no-volume practitioners on the medical staff, it is helpful to identify both strategic and competency goals, such as the following:

- Maintain strong relationships with the community's primary care base

- Protect against competitor encroachment by promoting practitioner loyalty

- Maintain a practitioner-friendly hospital culture

- Serve as a flexible partner for practitioners

- Maintain and grow market share through referrals

Although hospitals should maintain positive relationships with low- and no-volume practitioners, they should also maintain high credentialing and appointment standards. Goals related to ensuring practitioner competency include:

- Protect patients

- Grant practitioners privileges only for demonstrated competency

- Meet regulatory requirements

- Protect the hospital's reputation

Remember: Many primary care practitioners and specialty care practitioners who are ambulatory-based or non-hospital-based are a huge referral source (both for ancillary services and elected procedures) to hospital-based practitioners. By choosing not to allow low- and no-volume practitioners on the medical staff, the medical staff may disenfranchise this important referral source. Although low- and no-volume practitioners may not provide much or any care at the facility, medical staff leaders should carefully consider prohibiting them from voting, serving in office, or serving on committees, as they may still have valuable insight.

Hospitals should be physician-friendly and flexible partners for practitioners. They also want to maintain and grow market share. Therefore, although it is critical to establish competency standards and ensure that only competent practitioners are eligible to request privileges in the hospital, hospitals should also have strategic relationships with non-hospital-based practitioners.

Separate membership from privileges

In light of the strategic goals associated with having low- and no-volume practitioners on the medical staff, it is helpful to remember credentialing principle #12: Do not confuse membership and privileges. Membership categories determine the political rights a practitioner has as a member of the medical staff, which include the right to hold office, vote, constitute a quorum, amend bylaws, hold a meeting with the medical executive committee (MEC), and recall an election. Privileges determine what the practitioner can do as either a member or nonmember of the medical staff when providing patient care.

Most medical staffs find that four categories of membership work well:

- Active

- Associate

- Affiliate

- Honorary or emeritus

A practitioner in the active category is granted full political rights, including the right to vote and hold office. In the past,

Figure 6.1   MEDICAL STAFF MEMBERSHIP CATEGORIES

Membership category	Political rights of membership	Privileges allowed
Active	Full	Based upon provider's practice
Associate	Partial	Based upon provider's practice
Affiliate	Partial	Refer and follow
Honorary/ emeritus	Partial	Refer and follow or none

organizations typically gave active staff membership only to practitioners who had sufficient patient volume to exercise full independent privileges (more on the connection between patient volume and privileges later). Increasingly, organizations can be more flexible in this approach by giving low-volume practitioners the opportunity to be politically involved in the medical staff. Figure 6.1 gives examples of medical staff membership categories and privileges.

The associate category is for new members of the medical staff or those who don't meet a critical volume threshold. Again, the privileges allowed would be based on a provider's practice. Typically, associate members are not permitted to hold office, and they are often not permitted to vote in elections.

Traditionally, practitioners in the affiliate category were not granted privileges, but many hospitals are now granting these individuals refer-and-follow privileges. Refer-and-follow privileges allow a practitioner to refer a patient to the hospital, follow the patient in the hospital, and have access to federally protected information under the Health Insurance Portability and Accountability Act of 1996, but practitioners may not write notes or orders in the patient's chart.

Practitioners in the honorary or emeritus category typically have partial political rights and may have refer-and-follow or no privileges based on whether they continue to see patients. In terms of their political rights, the medical staff will need to exercise its judgment as to whether it would like these individuals involved in medical staff committees, as they have greater flexibility and time in their lives.

Privilege delineation concerns

In terms of competency, there are two types of low- and no-volume practitioners. There are those with adequate quality data elsewhere, such as another hospital or a freestanding surgical or ambulatory center. The credentials committee must examine that data to determine whether it answers the competency question adequately. The practitioner may be exercising different privileges at those other organizations than he or she is asking for at your organization and, therefore, the credentials committee must take a different route. For example, it may require that the practitioner be proctored during the first 12 procedures or it may grant the practitioner dependent privileges, meaning a fully privileged medical staff member must approve the low-volume practitioner's care plans.

The second category includes practitioners with inadequate performance data over the past 12–24 months, including physicians who may be reducing their scope of practice, returning from a leave of absence, or returning from early retirement.

If a practitioner has only done a procedure three times, there is insufficient quality data to determine his or her competence. He or she may indeed be fully competent, but the credentials committee needs further information. Joint Commission–accredited organizations are required to conduct focused professional practice evaluation (FPPE) to confirm a low-volume practitioner's competence, but it is also best practice for hospitals that are not accredited by The Joint Commission.

The key to successfully maintaining low-volume practitioners on the medical staff is to create gradations in privilege delineations. In the past, organizations typically granted practitioners either independent privileges or no privileges at all. Today, given the growing number of low- and no-volume practitioners, organizations must now create shades of gray. Medical staffs may wish to consider offering levels of privileges, such as the following:

- Independent

- Comanagement until proctoring/FPPE demonstrates competence

- Comanagement with hospitalist or other practitioner for the duration of privileging tenure (unlikely to generate necessary quality data)

- Dependent, typically held by allied health professionals

- Refer-and-follow

- None

If a practitioner only has three patient contacts a year, the credentials committee and the department chair can sit down with the practitioner and explain that he or she is not eligible for independent privileges, but the medical staff can offer dependent or refer-and-follow privileges. Offering a different level of privileges may help save the hospital's relationship with the practitioner while still acting in the best interest of patient care.

Which type of privileges is appropriate for each practitioner?

When determining whether the medical staff should grant a practitioner independent, comanagement, dependent, refer-and-follow, or no privileges, consider the following questions:

1. Is the practitioner licensed?

2. Is the practitioner authorized to practice independently in the institution?

3. Does the medical staff currently have adequate quality data/references to determine the practitioner's competency?

4. Is the medical staff likely to generate adequate quality data sometime in the near future?

If the answer to all four questions is yes, the candidate is eligible for independent privileges. If the practitioner currently does not have adequate quality data, the medical staff might want to

Figure 6.2

DETERMINING PRIVILEGE LEVEL

Privilege level	Licensed independent practitioner	Authorized to practice independently in the institution	Adequate quality data and/or references to determine competency	Likely to generate adequate quality data in the near future
Independent	Yes	Yes	Yes	NA
Comanagement until precepting demonstrates competence	Yes	Yes	No	Yes
Comanagement	Yes	Yes	No	No
Dependent	Yes or No	No	NA	NA
Refer and follow	Yes or No	No	NA	NA

     CREDENTIALS COMMITTEE ESSENTIALS HANDBOOK

consider the practitioner for comanagement privileges until proctoring demonstrates competence. If the medical staff does not have adequate, current quality data and it is unlikely to ever get it, the medical staff may just want to consider the practitioner for comanagement privileges. Finally, if the medical staff does not have any quality data, then the practitioner should only be eligible for dependent or refer-and-follow privileges. Figure 6.2 shows the different levels of privileges.

Impaired Practitioners

The American Medical Association states that a physician is impaired when he or she is unable to safely perform granted clinical privileges because of physical, emotional, mental, or personality issues, including deterioration through the aging process, loss of motor skill, and excessive use or abuse of drugs, including alcohol.

Medical staffs should not wait for a potential impairment to surface before creating a policy to deal with it. People are talented at hiding their impairments or addictions, so a physician who seems "normal" today may be the biggest problem on the medical staff's hands tomorrow. The medical staff should not try to deal with something as emotionally, politically, and economically charged as impairment without having a clear policy to follow. Elements of a good impairment policy and procedure include:

- Focus on protecting patients from harm

- Balance between patient protection and physician rights

- Approaching the practitioner with the goal of offering assistance and rehabilitation, not discipline

- Requiring the medical staff to look into and resolve concerns raised by anyone in the hospital involving potential impairment

- Creating a confidential process for investigating and resolving impairment concerns

The medical staff's goal should be to support impaired practitioners and help them exercise their privileges safely. Clearly, if a practitioner is actively using illegal drugs, the medical staff should prevent the practitioner from exercising privileges until he or she is clean, but a practitioner with a physical impairment, such as shaking hands, may simply need modified privileges. Typically, concerns should be resolved through a practitioner health committee or a practitioner advocacy committee, which may be a subcommittee of the credentials committee or MEC.

What is the role of the credentials committee when dealing with impairment?

The credentials committee develops the policy, procedure, and process by which it will evaluate potentially impaired practitioners. The credentials committee may also:

- Participate in continuous improvement of the practitioner health policy

- Refer identified concerns to the practitioner health committee

- Based on policy, assume primary responsibility if no practitioner health committee exists (or the MEC will assume this responsibility)

- Recommend status of the practitioner's privileges to the MEC after reviewing department chair recommendation

Aging Practitioners

The aging practitioner presents challenges that the medical profession has not addressed well in the past. The aging practitioner may be a beloved member of the medical staff with years of experience, who may or may not be exhibiting signs and symptoms of potential impairment. The question is whether the medical staff wants to wait for the impairment to manifest or identify potential impairment before it occurs.

Something as psychologically, emotionally, and politically charged as aging physicians requires a good policy and procedure that determines:

- The age at which the appointment cycle shortens, typically from two years to one year, and the practitioner is required to participate in an annual "fitness for work evaluation" annually (typically between ages 65 and 70)

- The age at which the practitioner is encouraged to move to ambulatory-based privileges (typically between ages 70 and 80)

- The age at which the practitioner automatically moves to honorary status (typically between ages 75 and 85)

A "fitness for work evaluation" is different than a physical examination in that it specifically addresses the physical, psychological, and cognitive issues that may preclude someone from exercising his or her privileges safely. The medical staff should include in its bylaws, policies, and procedures a stipulation that when a practitioner automatically moves to honorary status, typically between the ages of 75 and 85, he or she is not allowed procedure rights. The change in medical staff category is an administrative action and not a form of corrective action (corrective actions typically trigger the practitioner's right to a fair hearing and appeal).

If the medical staff does not already have a process for managing aging practitioners, then it will go through a period of growing pains, otherwise known as change management. Chances are, older practitioners on staff will resist the assumption that because they are in their golden years they can no longer practice safely. This is a very sensitive issue, so the credentials committee will probably want to go slowly and start by educating the medical staff about the effects of aging on the mind and body. Some credentials committees may wish to take a conservative approach by setting higher age limits in their policies and procedures. For example, the credentials committee may not shorten the reappointment cycle or ask physicians to participate in a fitness-for-work evaluation until age 70, rather than age 65.

To keep the process of evaluating aging practitioners objective, medical staffs may wish to contract with practitioners or organizations that do this work professionally.

Modifying the medical staff's approach over time and including a phase-in period may be the gentlest approach. Remember, these are some of the medical staff's most loyal and dedicated practitioners, and they deserve respect and dignity.

Privileging Disputes

An all-too-common challenge that medical staffs face is privileging disputes. Many medical staffs refer to these issues as *turf battles*, but that term implies an unprofessional approach to disagreements among physician peers. Rather than take a Sharks versus Jets approach to privileges, medical staffs must learn to manage privileging disputes in a fair and consistent way. The credentials committee typically handles privileging disputes because it can act as a referee if department chairs or section chiefs disagree.

Primary drivers of privileging disputes include:

- Money (declining incomes coupled with rising overhead)

- Technology (shorter learning curve reduces barriers)

- Exclusive contracts (is allowing only contracted physicians to perform specific privileges fair or unfair?)

- Overall sense of loss of control (anger)

Money. Perhaps the biggest driver of privileging disputes is money. Physicians feel squeezed as overhead rises and reimbursement decreases, and they are looking for additional revenue. Physicians can make more money not by seeing more patients, but by doing procedures. Because reimbursement is headed in the direction of procedures, physicians feel protective of their procedural privileges.

Technology. As technology evolves in a way that allows physicians to do the same procedures with a shorter learning curve, there are fewer barriers when it comes to obtaining privileges. Minimally invasive technology allows physicians to become competent performing a procedure quickly by taking a brief course to gain the necessary skills. The question then becomes "How much competence is enough?" The competence question creates a gray area that makes privileging disputes difficult to figure out.

Exclusive contracts. What if an exclusive contract covers a service that one of your physicians might become competent in? Interventional radiology and endovascular procedures are common examples of privileging disputes involving exclusive contracts. Take, for example, the cardiologist who says, "I can use a catheter in the coronary artery, so how hard can it be to do a peripheral artery in the leg?" The cardiologist wants to take a course and perform that procedure, but the radiologists refuse because endovascular radiologists have an exclusive contract to perform that procedure. The problem occurs when someone, typically a cardiologist or the largest cardiology group, expresses to management that although the procedure has been carved out in an exclusive contract, they would like to perform that procedure. Practitioners may pressure hospital administration by noting how much their department contributes to the hospital, and then the hospital must decide whether keep the endovascular privileges exclusive.

Overall sense of loss of control. Decades ago, practitioners called the shots. They decided how their practices would operate, but today, the government, payers, and hospital administration create narrow parameters within which physicians must practice. Physicians may feel frustrated that the hospital is determining whether they can get the training they need to perform procedures they want to do and whether they can earn additional income. When emotions run high, privileging disputes become turf battles.

The best approach to addressing privileging disputes is through a privileging dispute-resolution policy, which details the following step-by-step process.

1. Remember the four steps of credentialing (see Chapter 1). Don't tackle privileging disputes one at a time and try to invent a method to deal with each one. Figure out what your standard operating procedure will be to address privileging disputes and follow that consistently.

2. Establish a moratorium until the medical staff adopts a privilege dispute-resolution policy. If the medical staff

does not have a policy, stop and do not process a single privilege request until the credentials committee has created a policy.

3.   The credentials committee gathers information about the privileges under dispute by querying other organizations and reading literature on the subject. Here's the challenge: There is no national standard for privileging criteria. That's why each hospital and medical staff must develop its own. The task force meets and examines the various perspectives.

4.   Solicit recommendations from department chairs and other subject-matter experts. If they agree, you're done.

5.   If department chairs and other subject-matter experts do not agree, the credentials committee appoints a task force to develop criteria. The task force should be chaired by a member of the credentials committee who does not have a dog in this fight and is not part of the specialty that is disputing privileges. Do not just include representatives of the involved specialties on the task force, because they are not likely to remain objective. You need enough thoughtful third parties to resolve privileging disputes.

6.   The task force gathers additional information and makes a recommendation to the credentials committee

(sometimes with a minority report). If a practitioner applies for privileges that other practitioners claim are within their specialty, the medical staff policy should state that the credentials committee gathers recommendations from the department chairs or section chiefs and conducts extensive research.

7. The credentials committee reviews the task force's recommendation, deliberates, and recommends criteria to the medical executive committee (MEC), sometimes with a minority report. If, at this point, the representatives of the specialties involved in the dispute agree as to what the privileging criteria should be, you're done. Adopt the criteria, build them into the privilege delineation forms with eligibility criteria, and move on. Be sure to reference the medical staff's conflict-of-interest policy. If a member of the credentials committee is in one of the specialties involved in the privileging dispute, the medical staff must follow its conflict-of-interest policy to determine whether the committee member can participate in the discussion but refrain from voting, be removed from the discussion and voting entirely, or participate in the discussion and vote.

8. The MEC reviews the credentials committee's recommendation, deliberates, and recommends action to the governing board (sometimes with a minority report).

9. The governing board makes the final decision. If the privileging dispute is not too controversial and there is general agreement among members of the MEC, the MEC generally accepts the recommendation from the credentials committee. If there is deep division among members of the MEC, the issue is turned over to the governing board, which is the final conflict-resolving entity in the organization. The governing board takes all the input from the MEC, reviews the minority report, understands all the issues, and makes the final decision.

Using this step-by-step process, not everyone will be happy, but everyone will agree that the process is as fair and balanced as it can be. In today's healthcare environment, that's about as good as it's going to get.

The Credentials Committee's Role in Professional Conduct

The Joint Commission requires that medical staffs make evidence-based, objective decisions during both appointment and reappointment. Even if your facility is not Joint Commission–accredited, an objective, evidence-based process is best practice.

Credentials committees have to objectively assess a physician's competence based on not only on performance data, but also his or her professional conduct. Conduct is difficult to measure, and it is often politically charged.

As shown in figure 2.3 in Chapter 2, the medical executive committee (MEC) is responsible to the governing board to oversee and improve the professional competence and conduct of all practitioners granted clinical privileges. The credentials committee must take conduct issues into consideration when assessing a practitioner's qualifications for both membership and privileges on the organized medical staff. The peer review committee or quality committee may also have to take conduct into consideration with its performance measures, although the quality committee may defer that to the MEC and department chairs.

The organizational chart in the figure also shows that department chairs are accountable to the quality and credentials committees for their input and recommendations and for assessing practitioners' competency and conduct. When conduct concerns arise, the credentials committee should tap in to the department chairs for their assessments, evaluations, and recommendations.

How Does the Credentials Committee Handle Conduct Issues as Part of the Appointment and Reappointment Process?

The pyramid (see Chapter 2) offers a step-by-step process for evaluating the competence and conduct of practitioners on the medical staff. The base of the pyramid is to appoint excellent physicians (aka, credentialing and privileging), and the medical staff should have eligibility criteria for membership that includes character, ethics, and conduct. Including criteria about character, ethics, and conduct is important because it entitles the credentials committee to evaluate someone's conduct as part of both the appointment and reappointment process. This base layer of the pyramid acts as a filter; it should only allow capable, qualified practitioners onto the medical staff. If an unqualified candidate slips through, the medical staff must live with the decision until the next reappointment period.

The second layer of the pyramid is to set, communicate, and achieve buy-in to expectations. The credentials committee should have clearly articulated expectations regarding professional conduct, such as treating all individuals with respect and dignity at all times, even at times of disagreement.

To remind practitioners of the medical staff's expectations, the credentials committee should consider having practitioners sign a code of conduct policy as part of the reappointment process. If a practitioner displays disrespectful or disruptive behavior, he or she must read and sign the code of conduct as a reminder of the medical staff's expectation that practitioners act professionally. The code of conduct policy should state that in exchange for membership and privileges, practitioners agree to abide by the medical staff's bylaws, rules, regulations, policies, and procedures. If the practitioner refuses to sign the policy, he or she cannot be reappointed to the staff.

The next layer of the pyramid is to measure performance against expectations. Because professional conduct is important enough to consider for appointment and reappointment, medical staffs must come up with some feasible way to measure it. One way to measure professional conduct is through perception data, or how others perceive practitioner performance. There are two types of perception data: passive and active. Passive perception data includes data that was not solicited, such as incident reports, complaints, and compliments. Active perception data are data that the medical staff seeks from patients and other practitioners through focus groups, survey forms, and survey interviews.

The key is to balance subjective perception data with objective measures, such as the number of validated behavior incidences with targets for both excellence and adequate performance. The credentials committee can take these performance metrics into consideration at reappointment as part of the ongoing professional practice evaluation process.

Finally, the credentials committee should provide practitioners with periodic feedback in the form of feedback reports every six to eight months. Some of the quality metrics on that feedback report should address professional conduct, such as the number of validated staff complaints about practitioner communication or an average patient satisfaction percentile. Fortunately for the credentials committee, managing poor performance and taking corrective action is the purview of the department chairs, MEC, and governing board, but the credentials committee may wish to recommend corrective action to the MEC when a practitioner's conduct issues are so extreme as to preclude the safe exercise of granted clinical privileges.

Effective Credentials Committee Meetings

Does any medical staff member want to sit through one more meeting than necessary? Does any medical staff member want to sit through a meeting that's not using his or her time well? Credentialing is an important and fairly complex function that requires a committed and detail-oriented committee and organized, productive meetings. If committee members feel that meetings are unnecessary or a waste of time, their engagement may wane.

Following are five tips to create productive, effective meetings.

Tip #1: Provide for Appropriate Leadership and Membership

Following the pyramid model, selecting a chair and members of the credentials committee is much like selecting medical staff members during appointment and reappointment. The first step is to appoint excellent physicians or, in this case, excellent committee members. This process shouldn't be off the cuff—current committee members should vet new members thoroughly and speak to other medical staff members about the candidate's leadership skills, willingness to learn, and ability to work as part of a team.

To set, communicate, and achieve buy-in to goals, the medical staff should write a description of the responsibilities of the credentials committee as a whole, as well as the responsibilities of individual committee members. Consider what qualifications a practitioner should have to be eligible to serve as chair or member of the credentials committee. Will the medical staff require that members have past credentialing experience, or will it provide on-the-job training? Will the credentials committee provide new members with a crash course so that they can understand the committee's expectations up front and can jump right in to their responsibilities? Candidates must be interested in credentialing activities and willing to take the time to participate in training and become a vested committee member. Practitioners should not join the credentials committee to grind an ax for their particular specialty, they are there to be of service.

To measure performance, provide the committee chairs and members with job descriptions and measure how they perform in comparison to those descriptions. Finally, provide feedback to the credentials committee chair and members to give them an opportunity to improve.

To enable committee members to develop credentialing expertise, consider at least three-year terms on a rotating basis, so that each year, only one-third of the committee members change over.

Effective committee members should have the opportunity to sign on for a second term if they so desire. It takes a while to become a credentialing expert, especially when it comes to policies and procedures (that's the really thorny stuff). The credentials committee needs folks who understand credentialing, are invested in it, and stick around long enough to apply what they've learned.

The credentials committee is not representative of all specialties and departments, nor does it represent the interests of individual specialties and departments. It would be too cumbersome a group. The committee should focus on finding members who understand credentialing and are good at it and draw on appropriate subject-matter expertise for credentialing challenges when needed.

Tip #2: Spend Committee Time Wisely

Time is precious, so the credentials committee must spend it wisely. According to the four steps of credentialing (see Chapter 1), the credentials committee establishes policies and procedures (step one) and evaluates and recommends (step three). The credentials committee should spend time proportionately between those two activities. In that case, the committee must have enough time to deal with policy issues and create an efficient process for reviewing credentials files and making recommendations.

Usually, the credentials committee handles the process of delineating privileges and eligibility criteria and makes recommendations to the medical executive committee (MEC). The credentials committee has a lot of work to do in that space. Individual specialties may make recommendations to the credentials committee, but the credentials committee must make recommendations to the MEC about all of the aspects of privileging, particularly how to delineate privileges and what the eligibility criteria should be.

Given the credentials committee's responsibilities, the only way to find the time for work that doesn't relate specifically to credentialing and privileging recommendations is to:

- Have extra meetings (not very appealing)

- Structure committee activities so that only issues that warrant discussion are addressed by the full committee

- Consider an expedited process to focus attention on files with red flags

- Perform work routinely outside of committee meetings

The credentials committee meeting time should not be spent auditing files to check for the presence of routine information. If at the start of the credentialing committee meeting, each member is handed a stack of files to review, there is a problem with how the committee is organized to do its work. Members should review files before each meeting so that meeting can be spent tackling important issues.

Tip #3: Streamline Meetings by Eliminating Paper

The credentials committee should consider paperless means of completing its tasks. At a minimum, the committee can post agendas and related materials that members need to review prior to meetings on a secure website. Members can use an LCD projector at meetings to project the image of an application on the screen. A more technologically sophisticated approach involves electronic applications that members can review from their homes or offices at whatever time of day makes sense for them, without needing to go to the medical staff office during business hours.

Tip #4: Don't Forget Surveillance Activities

The credentials committee has the responsibility of being, in essence, the "antennae" of the organization. Members should research new issues, new technologies, and best practices for credentialing and privileging as the field evolves. Members should attend conferences, listen to audio conferences, read newsletters and publications, stay current with online postings, and discuss new ideas and best practices at meetings.

As developments occur, the committee should revisit existing policies and proactively develop new ones. Members may draft or modify a policy outside of a meeting, but the committee as a whole should review or rework the policy.

Tip #5: Provide Committee Support

Make sure your credentials committee has the kind of support it needs, including:

- **Knowledgeable and competent staff.** Medical staff services professionals can help the credentials committee accomplish its goals by taking meeting minutes, bringing credentialing developments to the committee's attention, organizing meeting times, and sending out reminders.

- **Sufficient resources.** Is the medical staff library well-stocked with credentialing resources, such as newsletters, books, and medical journals? Do committee members have online access to relevant databases? Are there enough funds for members to attend national conferences and other training opportunities?

- **Coordination and implementation of processes.**

- **Preparation of files for review, including identification of red flags.** Medical staff professionals are knowledgeable about credentialing and can flag issues in a medical staff application that need further attention. Credentials committee members should follow up on these red flags.

- **Identification of pertinent issues.** Do credentialing and privileging policies need updating? Are there privileging disputes raging between departments? The credentials committee must be able to identify these issues and act on them quickly.